Intermittent Fasting

4 Steps to Weight Loss, Muscle Growth, Energy Boost, and Body Auto-Healing Using the Proven Science of the Intermittent Fasting Lifestyle

By Faouez Khedhiri

Table Of Contents

About the Author

First, I want to say a very big "Thank you."

Not because you are reading this book, but for taking the first and right step to effect a change in your life just the same way I did.

My name is Faouez Khedhiri. I'm a certified sports nutrition coach who took the challenge and committed totally to change not only my body but my lifestyle and mindset.

I have always been into sports. When I was young, I played soccer for 10 years with my local team. Fitness and exercising were and still an important part of my life. In the other hand, dieting was not really important to me.

You must be wondering then why did I write this book and how did I get into this lifestyle. Well, I'm not going to claim a story of "I lost 20 pounds, that's why you have to follow my program".

My journey to this lifestyle that you will discover throughout the book, started with a tragic event. My uncle who passed away after suffering from diabetes for several years, and knowing my family history with this disease, were the major points in my life that made me reconsider the way I was living, eating and taking care of my health and body.

I started searching for diets that prevent diabetes and studying several training routines until one day, I watched a video of an online fitness blogger talking about intermittent fasting. I knew what fasting was all about considering the fact that I fasted before for religious reasons, but I had no idea what intermittent fasting is. So, I started to investigate and deeply studying this approach for 3 years. I was amazed by the facts and benefits that can occur from practicing this lifestyle.

Currently, I can proudly say that I'm on my way to upgrade my body, "a term that I love to use". I'm living a healthy and convenient lifestyle.

For that reason, I decided to make other people aware of this lifestyle, and I have coached several friends to achieve tremendous weight loss and health benefits.

As a next step, I decided to be more involved in the nutrition field. To achieve that, I got my certification as a sports nutrition coach and I wrote about this lifestyle that I follow to help someone who may be in need of such guides.

Everyone has that moment that makes her/him realize that **CHANGE** is necessary.

The start is crucial in any diet or lifestyle change and if you follow misleading or unproven information, your chances to continue are low.

Hence, the reason I will be sharing my journey and the 4 steps you need to ensure that the changes you make to your diet and lifestyle result in life-changing benefit.

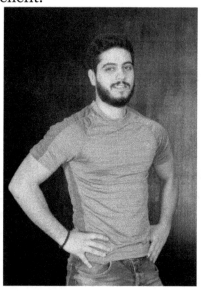

Join our community on Facebook:

"TRAINICS: Intermittent Fasting platform"

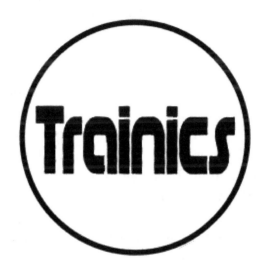

https://trainicsllc.wixsite.com/books

Introduction

One of the menaces in society today is excess fat. Many people do not live an active life. They typically engage in the same routine every day. Wake up, do a few chores, take the bus or train, or drive to work, come back from work, fix up dinner, curl up on the couch to watch TV, and sleep. The absence of exercise and lack of an active lifestyle contributes to packing excess fats. The food we eat also does not help. The grocery store is filled with bad carbs (pasta, starch vegetables, juice etc.) and fat-laden foods. All this adds to the body's fat storage.

In a bid to remedy this, there have been many weight loss diets that claim to help people lose weight. However, over time, many people have realized that these weight loss diets do not work. Traci Mann affirmed that while one might lose 5 to 10% of their body weight at first with a diet, it does come back. (Traci Mann, 2018). Many people are unable to abide by a weight loss diet because it restricts them to a particular food. Even some diet that do look promising would often mandate the user to work out like a maniac, in a bid to lose weight. And when they are lucky to get one that seems to work, there comes a time when they hit a plateau, or the weight comes back. This calls for a more sustainable approach to losing weight.

While many yoyo and fad diets will come and go, it has already dawned on many people that to lose weight, they need to reduce their calorie intake. That is why the most effective approach to weight loss is a healthy diet and lifestyle.

However, it is not that simple.

If you want to lose weight, your goal should be to burn more calories than you are consuming. The reverse also holds true if you want to gain weight. What you need to know is that those calories can't just come from anywhere. Calories are not all created equal. Even if you are burning the same amount of calories, the result of someone eating pizza and fast food will be different from one who concentrates on healthy meals. This brings me to macronutrients (Carbohydrates, Protein, Fat). Carbs are the body's energy source which gives the body four calories for every gram. The body breaks protein into amino acids after eating. However, unlike carbs, the body cannot store protein; hence it breaks it down for various uses. This is why the maximum daily consumption of protein is vital. Many people see fat as the bad guy. However, there are healthy fats that give out energy and help produce cholesterol in the body. (Cleveland Clinic, 2015, n.p). This is why you should focus strictly on healthy fats.

What is Ketosis?

To lose weight effectively, the best approach is to strive to get the body to a process called ketosis. When you get to ketosis, the body does not burn glucose for energy; instead, it turns on fat as its primary source of energy. Breaking down of fat in the body leads to the formation of ketones. A ketone is like an alternative to glucose which brings about fat loss. Ketones help in brain regeneration, improves heart disease, improve insulin sensitivity, aid in cancer therapy, etc. (Marjorie Hecht, 2018, n.p)

With intermittent fasting, you will get to ketosis. When the body gets to this state, you will start experiencing the advantages of fasting. Intermittent fasting, although primarily helps with weight loss, comes with a whole lot of other health benefits. Unlike many weight loss approaches, it stands out because it is not something you practice and then forget. It is a lifestyle that you have to grow into, which will make you enjoy the benefits when it becomes a lifestyle. This is why intermittent fasting stands out from many approaches to weight loss.

This is why you have this manual with you. This book will guide you as you grow into the IF (Intermittent Fasting) lifestyle.

Happy reading!

Chapter 1: What is Intermittent Fasting: History/ Definition

What is Intermittent Fasting?

While there are many different diet plans, one method that is often more effective at helping you work on your health and lose weight is intermittent fasting. This method can do so much for your body, and the ideas behind it are simple.

With intermittent fasting, you need to concentrate on eating healthy and wholesome foods, but there aren't strict requirements on the foods that you can and can't eat. With this option, you will focus more on separating your day into two periods, one for eating and one for fasting or abstaining from eating. The second time period, your fasting window, needs to be longer than normal to help better control your eating habits and the calories that you need to take in each day to improve your health.

Intermittent fasting and the different methods that go with it have grown in popularity. With all the great health benefits and the relative ease with which people lose weight on this eating plan, it is no wonder that everyone wants to give it a try. Let's take a look at some of the basics and history that you should know about intermittent fasting before moving on to discuss the benefits, how to get started, and so much more!

The History of Fasting

Fasting is not a new idea. It has been around for thousands of years. Pythagoras extolled the virtues of fasting, St. Catherine of Siena practiced fasting, and Paracelsus, a doctor during the Renaissance period, called fasting a "physician within" all of us. Fasting, in one form or another, is a distinguished tradition, and throughout the centuries, those who follow it claim that fasting can bring spiritual and physical renewal.

In primitive cultures, a fast would be needed before people went to war. It was also considered a coming of age ritual in many cultures. If the people were worried about an angry deity, a fast was often required, and North Americans would do it as a ceremony to avoid issues like famine.

Many of the major religions in the world have implemented fasting as part of their rituals. It can be used as a form of self-control and penitence or enacted for major events within the religion. For example, Judaism has several fasting days each year, including the Day of Atonement and Yom Kippur. In Islam, followers fast during the month of Ramadan. Greek Orthodox Christians and Roman Catholics will do a 40-day fast during Lent.

During the 19th century, a practice that was known as therapeutic fasting became popular to prevent illnesses and even treat some when they were done under medical supervision. This became something that grew with the Natural Hygiene Movement and is still popular today. This was seen as a natural way to help cleanse the body and prevent illnesses without having to worry so much about taking medicine that could cause many side effects and harm the body.

Today, there are many reasons why someone would choose to go on a fast. They may choose to do it as a part of their religion, or as a way to cleanse their bodies and help them lose weight. Fasting has a long history and many different uses, which makes it the perfect choice when you are ready to make some changes in your diet and lifestyle.

The Basics of an Intermittent Fast

Intermittent fasting is less about the foods that you eat – although these can be important – and more about the timing of your meals. With a traditional American diet, you can easily eat nonstop during the day. Many people start with breakfast, have a snack around midmorning, lunch, another snack, a big dinner, and even another snack before bedtime. There are even some healthy eating plans that recommend eating five or six times a day to help you lose weight.

What all these end up doing is allowing us to eat way too many calories during the day. We are feeding the body a constant supply of energy in the form of glucose, but most of it is not being used and is then stored as extra body fat over time. We get into a bad cycle of eating a bunch of bad carbs and calories, but still wanting more. This cycle is going to cause us to gain weight and possibly cause a whole host of other health conditions.

With intermittent fasting, you aim to change this cycle. You will learn how to limit your eating windows, not allowing yourself to eat all the time. This can help you reduce how much you take in and can naturally lead to weight loss. There are different options with intermittent fasting. Some recommend you to go 24 hours without eating, some recommend you to only eat 500 calories a few days a week, and others recommend you to do smaller fasts each day, limiting your eating window to eight hours or so.

No matter which method you choose to go with, you are limiting the amount of time that you can eat during the day. This results in fewer calories, easier weight loss, and more time to enjoy life. Think of all the freedom you will get just by cutting out a few of the meals that you have to plan and make each week!

There are different methods that you can choose when it comes to which type of intermittent fast you want. Some people like to go on an alternate day fast. Some like to do fasts a few days a week. Others like to have shorter fasts added into each day. All these methods can be effective; you just need to choose the one that fits into your schedule and stick with it.

Do I Need to Worry About Starvation Mode?

One common concern about intermittent fasting is that you will quickly put your body into starvation mode if you try this form of eating. The worry is that these small fasts are going to be enough to ruin one's metabolism and make it hard to lose weight or even function properly. The biggest issue here is that this concern is based on the idea that our bodies can't handle any stress, and going even a few hours without food can send it all out of order.

This is not true.

Think back to our ancestors. Did they have a constant stream of food at their disposal? Did they have horrible metabolic effects when they had to go a few days without eating because of famine or because the food was hard to come by? No, their bodies and ours were adapted to handle these shorter times without food to help them, and us, survive.

Starvation mode happens when you go a long time without food. The body starts to recognize that it isn't getting the nutrition that it needs, and so it will slow down your metabolism to keep you alive. However, studies show that it takes 72 hours or more before you start to see this occur. Intermittent fasting usually lasts less than 24 hours in a row. A few go up to 36 hours, but people usually cap it at that.

These fasts are not going to be long enough even to come close to the body going into starvation mode. Instead, during these short fasts, the body is going to spend time speeding up your metabolism, burning more calories as it goes through your readily available glucose and then moving on to Fat stores as well. Since the fast is so short, and with you concentrating on eating wholesome and nutritious foods during your eating windows, your body will burn more calories than normal, and there is no risk of entering starvation mode.

It is important that you stick with the fast that you chose and don't go overboard. If you don't eat healthy foods during your eating window, or you choose to eat too few calories during that time, and your fasts are too long, you could risk entering starvation mode and end up dealing with all the issues that come with that. However, if you follow your chosen intermittent fast well and you eat the right foods, you don't have to worry about this issue.

Chapter 2: Intermittent Fasting

Benefits

There are numerous benefits of intermittent fasting aside from the most obvious weight loss benefit. Below are some benefits of intermittent fasting that will keep your overall health in top shape.

Inhibition of Chronic Diseases

Chronic diseases such as diabetes and Alzheimer's Disease have been reported to have improved using intermittent fasting. Alzheimer's, in particular, is closely associated with obesity. This usually occurs in middle age when weight gain increases and abnormal proteins can become accumulated in the body. According to Dr. Jason Fung, renowned nephrologist and intermittent fasting expert, "It is believed that these abnormal proteins destroy the synaptic connections in the memory and cognition areas of the brain" (Fung, 2016, n.p.).

Chronic diseases usually result from insulin resistance. When your body functions optimally, the hormone insulin sends messages to your cells to extract glucose from your blood, and your cells act accordingly. But when cells in your liver, muscles, and other organs begin to ignore these messages, this is called insulin resistance. The human body is powered primarily by glucose. Developing a resistance to insulin means that your body is rejecting the very energy that powers it.

Insulin resistance causes glucose level or blood sugar level to increase significantly. This can be a precursor for type 2 diabetes. In addition, Non-Alcoholic Fatty Liver Disease (NAFLD) is a likely outcome of insulin resistance and this increases the likelihood of liver damage and contracting heart diseases (American Journal of Managed Care, 2013, n.p.).

Since fasting can result in a significant reduction in weight and the activation of a process that removes abnormal proteins, it can, in turn, have a positive impact in the treatment of obesity, diabetes, and Alzheimer disease.

Intermittent fasting also has a positive effect on combating adrenal stress or fatigue. Dr. Eric Berg aptly explains how the key to overcoming adrenal stress is the type of gradual eating adaptation that intermittent fasting provides. (Berg, 2019, n.p.).

Fat Loss and Weight Loss

When you are constantly consuming fewer amounts of calories (as intermittent fasting automatically compels you to), it is very likely that you will lose more weight and burn more fat. A review study conducted in 2014 strongly suggested that intermittent fasting can result in weight loss. Within a 3- to 24-week period, there was a significant 3 to 8% loss of body weight observed in participants who were made to fast intermittently for the duration of the study (Science Direct, 2014, p. 302-311). Another study strongly suggests that fat loss can result from fasting especially when combined with exercise (Mercola, 2013, n.p.).

Muscle Gain and Retention

Intermittent fasting promotes growth hormones which in turn maintain muscle during fasting. When intermittent fasting is combined with exercise, it has the effect of helping to gain and retain muscles. However, this would mean tweaking your meals to contain more carbohydrates. Equally, since gaining muscle is a direct function of exercising, you would have to increase the frequency of your workouts during fasting. (Fung, 2018)[9].

Note: Many people are arguing that Intermittent fasting is not for Muscle building. I have been fasting for 3 years and you can see the results yourself.

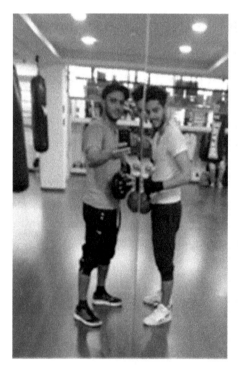

Before IF

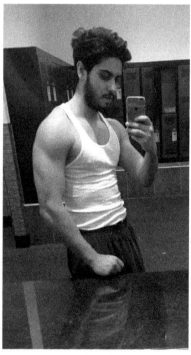

After IF

Convenience

Usually, with normal diets, when we wake up, we start thinking about what we will eat, and that is stressing, especially if you're in a hurry for work.

With intermittent fasting however, that isn't the case. Using this regimen, you don't really have to think about breakfast, nor do you have to prepare countless meals for the rest of your day. Generally, you don't even have to consider eating until your time window starts, so that is just one less thing on your mind.

Then again, even though the amount of food has to be controlled, as I will explain later on, intermittent fasting allows you to be very flexible with your food and enjoy big amounts of it.

In a nutshell, even though intermittent fasting obeys the laws of energy balance and is no magic, it is the perfect way to lose weight, while avoiding stress, remaining flexible, saving time and enjoying your food

Food enjoyment

Persisting hunger is one of the biggest issues of every person who has ever tried to lose weight. And it is no secret that basically every meal feels like a very tiny portion, which digests in no time and leaves you craving.

Well, while intermittent fasting does have physiological benefits, it also obeys the laws of energy balance and is no magic when it comes to weight loss. In other words, it works on the same principles as every other weight loss diet- You have to consume less calories than your daily energy expenditure to lose weight.

HOWEVER, the biggest benefit of intermittent fasting is that you can have HUGE meals. Especially if you get down to a shorter window of time, during which you can consume your food for the day.

And that is a really, really big psychological advantage- You get to consume massive amounts of food, but you also get to lose weight.

Pretty cool, isn't it?

Cellular Cleansing and Autophagy

New cells are produced in our bodies after old ones die off through a process called cellular cleansing. This automatic process that causes the new healthy cell to replace weak and worn-out ones can be stimulated by fasting.

Food intake causes a rise in our insulin levels and when we go without food, insulin levels, of course, drop. This drop-in insulin triggered by fasting also causes an increase in the hormone glucagon which helps to promote the cleansing of dead and worn-out cells. Damaged cells and irregular protein bodies are also removed from the body by a process called autophagy.

So, what exactly is that process we call autophagy? Well, the origin derives from Greek, where Auto means "self" and phagein means "eat", meaning that autophagy translates quite literally, to "self-consume".

Autophagy is basically the body's process, which removes the old, useless cells. In other words, we can refer to autophagy as a type of "Cellular recycling".

Dying cells may sound terrible, but we have to acknowledge the fact it is vital for sustaining good health. And this is exactly IF can again, be properly utilized to gain just one more benefit for the health.

That is to say that replacing old cells is not just related to general health, but can also improve certain diseases like cancer.

A small study with 10 cancer patients of different kinds (breast, prostate, lung), suggested that doing IF before and after chemotherapy can substantially reduce the side effects of that treatment. (Antunes, Fernanda, et al, 2018)

In another study, fasting, combined with platinum-based chemotherapy, promoted positive responses in most of the patients, affected by different stages of cancer. (Dorff, Tanya B, et al, 2016)

Other positive effects were the reduction of leukocyte DNA damage, as well as decreased levels of circulating IGF-1.

Both studies concluded that IF, when combined with cytotoxic agents is well-tolerated and safe for the majority of patients.

Bottom line is that fasting is not really magic for weight loss, but it certainly does have positive effects on other body systems, which, a regular diet would hardly produce.

Cognitive Function

The brain is the organ for cognitive function. When we are satiated, we have the tendency to want to relax or take a break from serious mental activities. On the other hand, when we are in a fasted state, our mental alacrity is sharpened. We tend to function optimally with less food in our stomach than when we are very full. Too much food has a way of dulling our brain alertness.

There have not been any studies to show that intermittent fasting negatively impacts brain function. On the contrary, fasting is known to boost reaction time, attention, sleep, mood, and other cognitive function.

Anti-aging

As we age, there is a decline in the production of growth hormone in our body. Bone mineral density is equally on the decline as we age. These, in combination with accumulated fat especially for those who do not have an active lifestyle, contribute to making us look and feel older than our actual age.

Fasting stimulates the production of growth hormones and increases the burning of stored fat. Equally, lean muscle is preserved when we make fasting a regular practice. All these can keep our bodies a youthful and allow us to age gracefully.

Now, let me explain how IF actually benefits that "graceful aging".

When it comes to anti-aging researches, calorie restriction and IF in particular have times and again been proven to be the most efficient means of doing so.

That is because calorie restriction benefits 5 main mechanisms that regulate healthy aging. (Moro, Tatiana et al., 2016)

Now, there are complex terms here, but we will list them out with their respective function

1. IGF-1 and mTOR- Associated with cell proliferation
2. NF-kB- Associated with inflammation
3. AMPK/SIRT- Associated with mitochondrial physiology
4. FoxO- Associated with autophagy
5. Nrf2- Associated with antioxidants

All of the mechanisms above are related to one another, meaning that aging, as a matter of fact is a complex process. So, it's not just time that passes by that makes you age, but also your lifestyle. Meaning that you can be at a certain astronomical age, but you can significantly improve your biological age, by improving your habits.

Bottom line- If you implement IF, you will hear "Wow, you look younger!" way more often, and you will be able to sustain that younger look and feeling for longer periods of time, ultimately, delaying your passing and making for a better quality of life.

Effects on Testosterone and Growth Hormone

There's a question that often pops up about intermittent fasting benefits, and it is namely about its effect on the endocrine system.

So, does IF boost the testosterone and growth hormone? Let's look at the facts, and help you optimize your hormonal levels.. Naturally.

Fact #1

For men of normal body-types, fasting increases the testosterone precursors by more than 50 percent and the overall testosterone concentration with nearly 200 percent. The study on this was not a long-term one, meaning that the affects were achieved quickly after starting the fast. (Röjdmark S., 1987)

Fact #2

Having lower body fat percentages allows your body to produce more testosterone. And while IF does not directly affect body fat as the energy balance does, it certainly is a good tool for burning body fat, as mentioned previously. (Harvard Health Publishing, 2011)

Fact #3

Major Growth hormone boosts. Another study shows that just within 24 hours of starting a fast, the body's growth hormone levels are elevated by as much as 5-fold. (Ho, K Y et al., 1988)

Now, considering that growth hormone and testosterone levels are correlated, not utilizing this tool, that intermittent fasting is, will make for a big miss.

Hunger management

Intermittent fasting has been proven times and again, to be a great tool for hunger management, and a regulator for other hormones, such as insulin and leptin.

Even though you might feel hunger from time to time, intermittent fasting regulates the hunger hormone called "ghrelin". What this means for you is that when you adhere to fasting, your hunger management will actually be BETTER. (Gotthardt, Juliet D et al., 2015)

Furthermore, with IF, your cognitive function will be greatly improved, making you literally laser-focused. That is mainly due to the improved levels of dopamine.

Last but not least, IF is an amazing tool for blood sugar regulation and the prevention of diseases like diabetes. Keep in mind though, transitioning to intermittent fasting should be done gradually, as to avoid subjecting the body to drastic changes. Remember, the body takes time to adapt, whether it is about training, nutrition or even adapting to a new time zone.

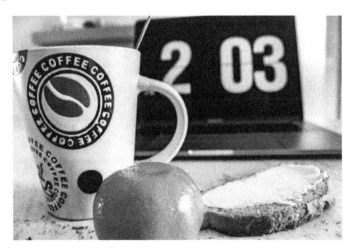

IF Regulates Gut Flora

There are many types of microbes in our bodies that have different functions. As a matter of fact, there is a big number of microbes in our guts that regulate digestion and can impact our health and hunger management. (Catterson, James H et al, 2018)

That is to say that we have to take care of those little guys inside of our guts, as they can quite literally change our health, for better or for worse.

Most people use IF for other benefits, but the gut-health benefit of it is often underestimated. Fasting favors the balance of beneficial gut bacteria, which protect against many metabolic diseases, such as the metabolic syndrome.

On top of that, as IF makes weight loss easier, that fat loss in turn accounts for better gut health DIRECTLY.

So, again, why wouldn't you include fasting a couple times a week? It's a win-win! You get to enjoy big amounts of food, you get to lose weight and you get to feel better and more energetic, with an improved gut function.

Furthermore, when you know you won't be consuming foods that are bad for the gut right before bedtime, you can rest assured that your gut will be a hundred percent healthy.

Eventually, you will lose the (delicious & bad) habit of eating gut-heavy foods before going to bed, which will ultimately improve your overall health and body composition.

Who Would Benefit the Most from Intermittent Fasting?

Almost everyone can benefit from going on an intermittent fast. It helps to speed up the metabolism, can give you more energy, puts the body in fat burning mode and often can result in weight loss and health benefits, unlike any other diet plan according to a study published in the Journal of Physiology. People who would benefit the most from starting an intermittent fast are:

- Those who want to lose weight

- Those who want to change their eating habits

- Weightlifters and bodybuilders

- Those who want to make life easier with fewer meals to plan

- Those who want to improve their heart health

- Those who want to help fight diabetes

- Those who are looking to keep the brain healthy and working well

- Those who are want to get rid of belly fat

Is There Anyone Who Shouldn't Go on an Intermittent Fast?

While an intermittent fast can be a great way to help improve your health and lose weight, some individuals should consider not doing an intermittent fast. These individuals may experience trouble getting the right amount of nutrition through the day when they fast, and they may have to worry about medication or other issues that fasting can aggravate. People who should consider not doing an intermittent fast, or at least should discuss it with their doctor ahead of time, include:

• Children and teenagers who are still developing and growing

• Women who are currently pregnant

• Women who are currently breastfeeding

• People who have recently had surgery and are recovering

• People with certain eating disorders

• Those who are severely underweight

• Those who are dealing with diabetes that is controlled with insulin

• Those taking medication - some types of medications can be negatively affected by an intermittent fast as well. Make sure to discuss this with your doctor before starting

Intermittent fasting is a great lifestyle that makes it easy for you to lose weight and improve your health. However, concerning the above conditions, it can be a challenge to fast regarding getting adequate nutrition throughout the day, and not just during short eating windows.

Chapter 3: Four Steps to Start Fasting

Step 1: Choose the best type of fasting to suits you

There is no right or wrong way to perform a fast. The rule of thumb is to not consume any calories for however long the fast lasts. This can be anywhere from a few hours when skipping a meal to over 24 hours when fasting for a day or longer. However, any fasting routine is only effective if it is sustainable for the long term. If the fast is too difficult to perform, then it does very little. The fast needs to be in conformance with the lifestyle of the practitioner both in terms of controlling appetite and providing ample energetic needs when needed. Thankfully, there are several different intermittent fasting routines to choose from. These are suitable for beginners as well as for advanced fasters. It is not recommended that someone new to fasting pick a routine that is too difficult. If you are already burned out from faulty dieting, the last thing you need is an overbearing routine.

Fasting routines

Pick whichever you feel is a good start. With no prior fasting experience, it is difficult to gauge how well you will do. The easiest version of the fast is to simply skip breakfast and or lunch and eat whatever you want for the rest of the day. Do not be afraid of skipping meals. Most Americans have been drilled into their heads with the idea that breakfast is the most important meal of the day. This has little scientific basis other than the fact that it gives you more energy to start off the day. All meals are equally as important as each other. The problem with designating breakfast as the most important is that people tend to overeat simply for the sake of their meal being a "hearty" breakfast. People tend to load up on carbs during their breakfast meals. Cereal, bagels, doughnuts, muffins, and other sugary foods are all big no-no's. It is perfectly okay to skip breakfast. It will cause no harm to you. If you are overweight, skipping breakfast will only work in your favor by lowering the concentration of insulin.

Beginner's Fast # 1

Breakfast means literally to break a fast that you undergo from the night before. Every time you break a fast, you will want to introduce a small number of calories. Eating too much too soon can overload the liver. The ideal meal for breakfast is a small, high protein mix of veggies and meat that will keep you satiated for longer. Eggs and avocados are some of the best foods you can have. Throw in a piping hot cup of coffee or tea and you have a true breakfast of champions.

This beginner's fast consists of a small meal upon waking followed by a six- to eight-hour fast. The eating window starts immediately after those eight hours are up. Those who work a regular 9 to 5 job can simply eat a small breakfast in the morning and not eat until coming home from work.

Beginner's Fast # 2

This fast consists of an eight-hour fast overnight followed by another four hours of no eating upon waking. Eat a small meal before going to sleep and follow it up with a small meal to break the fast. This probably means that you will miss both breakfast and lunch, but that is okay. Your eating window will begin somewhere in the mid-afternoon depending on what time you wake up. This is a 12-hour fast which sounds daunting at first but isn't too hard for most people. You can probably recall times when you had to skip breakfast and lunch for whatever reason. It was probably difficult, but it wasn't the end of the world.

Skipping breakfast and lunch means you may go into work feeling a little out of sorts. Drink plenty of water and caffeinate as needed. You will only have to worry about four hours of hunger pangs before being able to eat again.

The 16/8 Method

This routine is pretty straightforward. You fast for 16 hours every day and enjoy an 8-hour eating window. The fast technically begins after your last meal the day before. If your last meal is at 6 PM, you can eat again at 10 AM. For most, this is a very flexible plan. You can begin your fasting period the day before earlier or later. This will allow you to schedule important outings with family and friends away from the fasting period. Eating breakfast at 10AM is also common for many people.

This method is also known as the Leangains protocol, and was popularized by fitness expert Martin Berkhan.

Note that the fasting period and eating window add up to 24 hours. The fasting scheme can increase in difficulty by simply moving these numbers around. Following 16/8, the next logical progression is 18/6, 20/4, and so on. This routine is not recommended for beginners and should be worked up to from the beginner routines.

The Warrior Method

Hunters and militiamen in the past worked or trained all day and then came home to eat. In times of war, victories were rewarded by extravagant feasts. The warrior diet attempts to mimic the eating habits of those who went through periods of famine and feast. The warrior diet was popularized by fitness expert Ori Hofmekler. The rules are to fast for the entire day and eat a large meal at night. As you can imagine, the eating window is very small here, anywhere from 2 to 3 hours.

As always, break the fast with a small meal, wait for 45 minutes to an hour and then dig in. The meal should be larger than average and should be high in protein and fats. If this meal is high in carbohydrates, then blood sugar may spike. Limit how many carbs you eat!

24-Hour Fasts and Beyond

Fasting for up to 24 hours is usually what comes to mind when people say "fasting". It usually takes around 24 hours for the body to use up all of its glycogen stores and begin to tap into fat. The depletion can be accelerated by low-carb diets and exercise. After 24 hours, blood sugar may paradoxically rise as the liver tries to create a little extra glucose from amino acids and glycerol. Any rise in blood sugar at this stage must be endogenous because you haven't consumed any calories. Soon, this glucose will also run out and ketone bodies will begin to produce. Somewhere along this journey, you will also experience a strange increase in available energy. As the body transitions to running on fat, you will be much more energetic than in your glucose-energy deprived state.

Eat-Stop-Eat is a method that involves a 24-hour fast, either once or twice per week. This method was popularized by fitness expert Brad Pilon, and has been quite popular for a few years.

Beyond 24 hours, hunger pangs should go down as well. If you have ample fat stores to begin with, you won't feel as hungry while in ketosis. A beginner faster or someone with a diet that is high in carbohydrates and sugar will struggle to get into ketosis from just fasting. For them, fasting for 24 hours is much more difficult as the body needs to burn more sugar before it gets to ketosis. It takes time for the liver to detoxify from sugar as well. But the more you become adapted to burn fat, the quicker you can enter into ketosis.

Keep hydrated and take a daily multivitamin if needed. Drink mineral water to replenish sodium and or prepare a bone broth. If at any time you experience diarrhea or excessive vomiting, then immediately end the fast. If you experience lightheadedness, dizziness, nausea, or loss of consciousness, end the fast and seek medical assistance if necessary.

Step 2: Know what you can consume during a fast

In addition to different routines, each can be modified to suit the personal preferences of the person. A fast should be strict, but it should also be accommodating enough that it can be done several times a week for months at a time. Going for long periods of time without eating anything is not easy. The trick is to make it easy wherever possible. The intermittent fasting standard is to avoid all caloric consumption and to only drink water. It is not recommended to forgo a fast without staying hydrated throughout. As the old saying goes, you can live for months without eating but only a few days without water. Just plain water is zero calories. This includes the array of bottled water brands purchasable at any grocery store. Mineral water, sparkling water, club sodas, and other zero calorie drinks are also permitted. Coffee and all different varieties of teas are also fasting favorites.

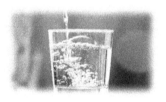

Water is straightforward, but concerns begin with adding anything to it. Water additives that contain sugar are not allowed under the intermittent fasting standard. This means no Kool-Aid, sports drink mixes, or protein shakes. No soda of any kind is allowed. Some fasters like to indulge in the occasional diet soda drink on their fasts. While diet soda sports a label with "zero calories," these drinks are not recommended if long-term weight loss is the goal. Black coffee is the preferred option, but many do not like it. In that case, Coffee can be sweetened with natural herbs and spices like cinnamon, chai, and nutmeg. Do whatever you can do to make the fast enjoyable but keep in mind that calories are supposed to be eliminated.

In fact, black coffee is a powerful tool that has some effect on autophagy, which means it can speed up the process of cell recycling. According to research published in Cell Cycle Journal, Polyphenols in coffee encourages cells to undergo autophagy much more than those that did not consume coffee.

Loss of sodium is common on longer fasts and a good option is to replenish sodium levels is by eating bone broths. This is easy to prepare and animal bones are relatively inexpensive from butcher shops and specialty food stores. Beef, chicken, and even fish bones are all suitable for broths. Bones that contain more meat tend to make for a higher calorie broth but there isn't much difference. Broths can be prepared with other spices for taste, as well as cuts of vegetables. They can be enjoyed hot or cold.

A good beginning fasting routine is one that allows you to perform the fast until completion and works well with your cravings. Your ability to resist cravings will strengthen with time. You should program two to three days a week for fasting. Note that this doesn't mean you will be fasting for the entire day or even close to it. Every night, you should be receiving anywhere from 6 to 8 hours of sleep. Time spent in bed technically counts towards your fast. A twelve-hour fast then may consist of 8 hours of sleep and 4 hours upon waking. The same can be said when you eat your last meal in the evening and don't consume any additional calories until the next time. Longer fasts will seem less daunting with the knowledge that you can start the day before.

Once in your eating window, there are no restrictions on calorie consumption besides the ones prescribed by objectives you are seeking. It's important that you count calories. BUT DO NOT OVER THINK IT! Your objective of losing or gaining weight will dictate your calories needed. Note that fasting is not an excuse for gorging on all-you-can-eat buffets. You won't lose any weight this way. At the end of the day, fasting is merely a tool for regulating your blood sugar and insulin levels. Diabetics and others who have pre-existing conditions will need to talk with their doctors before making any significant changes to their eating habits.

When Should I Fast?

In general, it is recommended to have 2 to 3 fasting days a week for weight loss. This can include any combination of the above fasting methods. Some prefer longer fasts with fewer days a week and others prefer shorter fasts more times a week. Some intermediate variations include two 24-hour fasts a week, three 16-hour fasts a week, or alternate day 24-hour fasts. The beginner fasts are suitable for high frequency and can even be done up to 7 days a week.

> Note: When I first started, 3 years ago, I began with 12hours of fasting. Then, I started to increase my fasting time, gradually. Currently, I fast 16 to 18 hours, every day, including 8 hours of sleep.

These decisions will be up to you and your commitments. The ideal fasting day is one where you can keep busy to get your mind off food but that also puts you somewhere away from food. Scheduling a fast on days when you have lunches planned, holidays, celebrations, and other social outings is a bad idea. Even walking by a cafeteria or place that exudes the aroma of cooked food can be enough to give in to cravings.

Step 3: How to break your fast

Bear in mind that for you to get the full benefits of intermittent fasting, it is not all about starvation. You must know how to break your fast. This includes being smart with your choice of food and drinks.

Whatever your reason for adopting intermittent fasting, you should strive to follow the right guidelines in breaking your fast.

This is because fasting alters body metabolism as there are some hormonal changes during fasting. Some examples are increased luteinizing hormone, increased growth hormone, autophagy, and the like.

Fasting also puts you into the state of ketosis – the stage when the liver converts fatty acids into ketones. However, bear in mind that during fasting, the body has already adapted to the absence of food, hence a pause in the digestive system. As a result, you cannot just eat whatever you like. You do not want to trigger inflammation or stress your digestive system.

How to break your fast

In breaking the fast, you need a food item that stimulates the digestive system without releasing insulin. A perfect food choice is apple cider vinegar. This is because it is known to balance pH levels, give stable blood sugar levels, and gets rid of harmful gut bacteria. (Yuri Elkaim, n.p). You can include lemon due to the citric acid content as it activates digestive enzymes before eating.

Before you Eat, Know your Calorie Intake

As living beings, we need a certain amount of energy to maintain the body's mass in space. For us humans, that energy is referred to as "Calories" and comes from food.

That is to say that we need a certain amount of food not only to maintain our bodyweight, but also maintain proper functioning of all physiological processes in the body.

That is exactly why, a weight loss diet should not be taken to the extremes, as you want to lose the weight in a healthy manner. A proper weight loss period is one, during which we managed to lose weight, but also kept our energy levels normal, rather than reaching excessive exhaustion.

So, knowing this, the first thing we have to do is be aware of our daily energy expenditure- How much energy our body burns daily, to maintain its weight.

Factors determining Daily energy expenditure

That number of calories is referred to as "Total daily energy expenditure" or shortly, "TDEE".

The TDEE depends on a number of factors-

- Gender
- Age
- Height
- Weight
- Exercise output

Activity levels (Outside of training, for example- Is your work sedentary, such as an office job, or is it moderately/highly active, such as a teacher or food delivery with a bike?)

All these factors account for the majority of your TDEE, and are calculated with certain formulas, which I will show you in a bit.

Steps to Calculating Your Daily Calorie Needs

Step 1: Find out t your weight in kilograms. Divide your weight in pounds by 2.2 if you live in the US or Canada.

Step 2: Multiply your weight (in kg) by 1.0 for men and 0.9 for women.

Step 3: Multiply that number by 24.

Step 4: Multiply the value you have by the value of your Lean Factor from the table below.

	Body Fat Percentage	Lean Factor Multiplier
Male	10 – 14	1.0
	15 – 20	0.95
	21 – 28	0.90
	Over 28	0.85
Female	14 – 18	1.0
	19 – 28	0.95
	29 – 38	0.90
	Over 38	0.85

Table Source: https://diabetesstrong.com/how-to-find-your-daily-calorie-need/

This is known as the Basal Metabolic Rate (BMR). The basal metabolic rate is the amount of calories you burn in a day without any dangerous activity. However, we need specifics. You need a specific value for the number of calories you would consume each day. To get this value, multiply the value you got above by your "Activity Modifier."

Daily Activity level Multiplier
1.3 (very Light Activity) – Normal office job (typing, sitting and studying with little walking in a day)
1.55 (Light) Jobs requiring you to stand or walk about (teaching, lecturing, shop, laboratory work, etc.)
1.65 (Moderate) Any job requiring some level of physical activity (cleaning, biking, jogging, maintenance or working out 2 hours per day)
1.80 (Heavy) heavy manual labor (Dancer, construction, carpentry, athlete, etc, and general hard physical activities, 4 hours per day)
2.0 (Really Heavy) Moderate to hard physical activity, about 8 hours per day

Table Source: https://diabetesstrong.com/how-to-find-your-daily-calorie-need/

The final value you have is your TDEE (the amount of calories you need in a day) .

Example using my statistics:

70 kg (154.3 pounds) * 1.0 (male) * 24 * 1 (14% body fat) = 1680

My daily calorie need = 1680 (my BMR) *1.65 (Moderate activity) = 2772 calories per day

I found out my TDEE, now what?

Well, now you're a step closer to triggering weight loss, or muscle gain. As we cleared out, the TDEE is the amount of energy (calories) you need to MAINTAIN your bodyweight.

From then on, it is simple mathematics- Consuming less calories than your TDEE consistently, will lead to consistent weight loss. That is called being in a "Caloric deficit".

On the flipside, consuming more calories than your TDEE will lead to consistent weight gain. That is called being in a "Caloric surplus".

Logically, consuming just the same as your TDEE, will lead to no progressive increases or decreases in weight. Simple as that.

Now that you know the principles of weight control, you can calculate the TDEE & daily macros, using my guidelines below.

Calculate Your Macronutrient Needs

Calories differ and are not created equal. You need to understand that some calories are much crucial than others. You will be much better off eating 100 calories from beans and nuts, compared to 100 calories from pizza, potato chips, and giant donuts.

Many health practitioners and fitness experts have advised that protein is essential for prompt recovery after a workout. (Arlene Semeco, 2016, n.p). It is because protein provides better calories, and fosters muscle growth while keeping you full.

Carbs also provide the necessary energy for optimum performance for a workout.

With fat, you get healthy skin and hair, and condition your body to absorb food nutrients better

Be smart about your choice of food when breaking your intermittent fast. Do not be so fixated on calories alone, as you have got to know how to get it right with the macronutrients as well – carbs, protein, and fat.

How do you go about getting it right with your macros?

Protein Intake

If you want to lose weight, you need to concentrate on 1 to 1.2 grams of protein for every single pound of body weight. This will give you an optimum result.

Consider 1 gram of protein per pound of your body mass if you are already overweight. By overweight, we mean 30% body fat for female and 25% body fat for a male.

To gain or maintain your body weight, be sure to concentrate on a gram of protein per pound of body weight in your meals per day.

For fat intake

Concentrate on 0.2 to 0.25 grams of fat per pound of your body weight per day, if you aim to lose weight

To maintain your body weight or gain muscle, focus on 0.3 to 0.36 grams per pound of your body weight.

On a final note:

- your daily carb intake should usually be between 30 to 35% of the overall calories needed in a day.

- Protein intake should be between 40 to 50%

- Fat intake should be around 20 to 25%

Have you ever tried recording your activities on a daily basis? What do you eat? When do you eat? How many hours of sleep? How many hours of fasting?

You'd be surprised at what it can reveal about your Lifestyle habits. A food log is an excellent option to track your calories and Macros intake.

Visit **http://bit.ly/2TY3tny**

to get your **FREE BONUS** of Free world page food log.

My Name:		Date:	
	Summary	Time	Food Type
Start of Fasting			
Start of Eating window			
First Meal			☐ Homemade
			☐ Package
			☐ Outside
Second Meal			☐ Homemade
			☐ Package
			☐ Outside
Third Meal			☐ Homemade
			☐ Package
			☐ Outside
			☐ Package
			☐ Outside
			☐ Package
			☐ Outside
Water Intake			

Total			
Calories	Protein	FAT	Carbs

What to Eat When Breaking a Fast

(Break your fast Without Coming out of Ketosis)

Medium Chain Triglyceride (MCT) are quickly absorbed into the bloodstream (Nutrition Review, 2013, n.p); hence, releasing energy fast. So we advise taking some MCT oil to break your fast. This is a good thing because the fat burning process keeps going, helping you remain in ketosis for longer.

Be sure to wait for about 20 minutes after taking the lemon water and MCT oil. This is to give your intestine enough time to absorb the nutrients.

You should feel your intestine waking up gradually, which is a good sign.

Generally, carbs will make you hold on to excess water weight. This is pronounced if you are taking them with excessive sodium and potassium. While a spike of insulin is good (because it helps the body cells absorb nutrients), there are some adverse effects as well like loss of sleep.

In this regard, your aim should be consuming minimal food which is low on the glycemic index. By doing this, you remain in a semi-fasted state and still get to enjoy the benefits of ketosis.

Some common examples include chickpeas, bananas, lentils, soy products, milk, pasta, grain bread, apples, berries, and pears.

What Should the Size of Your Meal be when Breaking?

Except if you chose the warrior diet type of intermittent fasting, be sure to start by eating something small. Warrior diet fasting is the intermittent fasting type that comes with a 4-hour eating window at night to eat a huge meal. This is one of the avenues while it is advisable to eat large meals.

Also, if you had worked out while fasting, you should be after protein synthesis. Hence, be sure to concentrate on more calories to foster the absorption of amino acids into your cells.

If you are not on any restrictive diet, which I prefer, be sure to include carbs. This will foster an insulin response that will help in muscle building, instead of fat. Choose healthy carbs such as potatoes, ripe bananas, and rice cakes.

For people on the keto diet, we recommend foods like eggs due to the high leucine content. Leucine is an amino acid that helps muscle growth.

The Ketogenic diet and Intermittent fasting share the benefit of making the body into Ketosis. For that reason, people are mixing these two approaches to maximize their results. In my opinion, since I followed the Keto diet before, this diet is optimal for the short-term. Good Carbs have an important role in our bodies as explained before.

Visit http://bit.ly/2TYtovx

and get everything you need about the Ketogenic diet, a 4 weeks meal plan, and the grocery list for the recipes!!

Note: Personally, I tried different diets like Keto and low-fat diets. My conclusion is that all these restrictive diets are not optimal. You may see results on the short-term but it will not be optimal for the long-term. Carbs, Fat, Protein are all important for our bodies and their functioning.

Step 4: How to Start and Adapt to Intermittent Fasting

One of the best things about intermittent fasting is that it is not restrictive. As discussed in the first step, there are many types of intermittent fasting. However, there is no specific method to determine the best fit for anyone. Necessity lies on you to listen to your body and learn the type of fast that works for you. The fact that your partner, friend, or co-worker attempted the 16/8 method and had a smooth ride doesn't mean that is the ideal for you.

As said earlier, intermittent fasting is a lifestyle. It takes practice, patience, and dedication to listen to your body to determine the most suited type for you. It is not a diet that you attempt for a couple of months and leave. It is a lifestyle that you need to grow into.

Irrespective of who you are and your age, intermittent fasting comes with obvious health benefits, too many to ignore.

How to get started with intermittent fasting

Many people dread the mention of the word 'fast' as it triggers an image of horrible suffering, inconvenience, and starvation. It is too much for some people even to imagine themselves going without food.

Fasting is not as bad as it sounds and doesn't have to be a painful experience. You can take a healthy approach to your fast, whatever the type of intermittent fast you chose to go with.

For instance, you had your last meal around 8 pm, and you hit the hay around 10 pm. Between this two-hour window, your body will be in a semi-fasted state. Assuming you had 8 hours of sleep, you have slept off a portion of your fasting window. It is a good idea to let a part of your fasting window fall during your bedtime. This is to renew your energy and keep you in top condition for the remaining duration of your fast.

Chances are you might not feel hungry in the morning, depending on the quantity and type of food you ate the night before. As you progress with the fast, be sure to drink water when the hunger pangs set in. Most times, the body interprets dehydration as hunger. Drink water and coffee (coffee without sugar) at an interval.

If you are new to fasting, it is best to start small. Be sure to listen to your body. When the hunger becomes unbearable, you can break following the step mentioned previously. Note the time you broke the fast. On your next fast day, be sure to push the time a little further. This is the best part of intermittent fasting. There is no one size fits all, and you grow into it.

All in all, you have got to be dedicated and highly disciplined to succeed with the fast. Many people have an unhealthy relationship with food. Many practice stress eating, emotional eating, etc. This makes it quite difficult to fast. This is where determination and self-discipline come in.

Fasting is not as hard as our subconscious interprets it to be. Deciding to fast is the start of a healthy relationship with food. Take that as time to reflect on the bad food choices you have made over the years. With fasting, you get to turn it around, build a new relationship with food, and also enjoy tremendous health benefits.

Food Choices during Fasting

On the last meal before the fast, be sure to stay away from foods that are hard to digest like hard meat. Limit dehydrating foods like crackers. Simple carbs like sugar and sweetened coffee are also not advised.

Sweet desserts will likely make you thirsty, stay away from them. After a couple of hours, it might lower your blood sugar level increasing your craving for sweets. (Body and Soul, 2013)

The best foods to eat before fasting are foods that take quite a while to cook. These are foods that have absorbed heat from cooking. They are foods that preserve energy as extended, and examples include legumes, beans, and soups rich in orange vegetables.

Fasting does not restrict you to a specific diet, but if you continue to take in too many calories and eat unhealthy food, you are going to have a hard time seeing results on your fast.

Recipes and Meal plan

GREEN PROTEIN SMOOTHIE

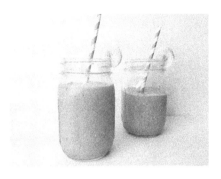

INGREDIENTS

1/2 Frozen Banana

1 Cup of Spinach

1/2 Avocado

1 Serving of Vanilla Protein Powder

1 Cup of Almond Milk

1 Tbsp of Chia Seeds

NUTRITIONAL VALUE

Fat: 20 g/ Carbs: 28 g/ Protein: 42 g

Total Calories: 430 Calories

DIRECTIONS

Start by pouring the almond milk into the blender to avoid the ingredients sticking at the bottom of the blender. Next add in the banana, avocado, spinach, chia seeds and the protein powder. Turn the blender on, starting at a low speed and increase as needed. Once the liquid looks even, pour into a cup and enjoy immediately to conserve as many nutrients as possible

RASPBERRY COCONUT SMOOTHIE

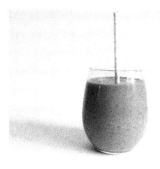

INGREDIENTS

1 Cup of Raspberries

1/2 Frozen Banana

1 Tbsp of Chia Seeds

1 Cup Coconut Milk

1 Serving of Vanilla Protein Powder

NUTRITIONAL VALUE

Fat: 10 g/ Carbs: 54 g/ Protein: 41 g

Total Calories: 448 Calories

DIRECTIONS

Start by pouring the coconut milk into the blender to avoid the ingredients sticking at the bottom of the blender. Next add in the banana, raspberries, chia seeds and the protein powder. Turn the blender on, starting at a low speed and increase as needed. Once the liquid looks even, pour into a cup and enjoy immediately to conserve as many nutrients as possible

BLUEBERRY SMOOTHIE

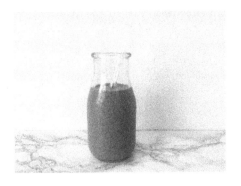

INGREDIENTS

1 Cup of Blueberries

1 Banana

1 Cup of Coconut Milk

1 Serving of Vanilla Protein Powder

Handful of Ice

NUTRITIONAL VALUE

Fat: 18 g/ Carbs: 53 g/ Protein: 20 g

Total Calories: 436 Calories

DIRECTIONS

Start by pouring the coconut milk into the blender to avoid the ingredients sticking at the bottom of the blender. Next, throw in the blueberries, banana, collagen powder and the ice. Turn the blender on, starting at a low speed and increase as needed. Once the liquid looks even, pour into a cup and enjoy immediately to conserve as many nutrients as possible.

CHOCOLATE BANANA SMOOTHIE

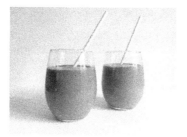

INGREDIENTS

1 Frozen Banana

1/2 Avocado

1 Cup of Almond Milk

2 Tbsp of Raw Cacao Powder

1 Serving Chocolate Protein Powder

NUTRITIONAL VALUE

Fat: 10 g/ Carbs: 54 g/ Protein: 41 g

Total Calories: 448 Calories

DIRECTIONS

Start by pouring the almond milk into the blender to avoid the ingredients sticking at the bottom of the blender. Next, throw in the banana, avocado, cacao powder and the protein powder. Turn the blender on, starting at a low speed and increase as needed. Once the liquid is even pour into a cup and enjoy immediately to conserve as many nutrients as possible.

SUPERFOOD OATMEAL

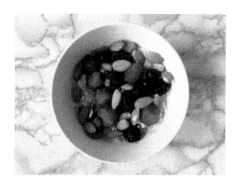

INGREDIENTS

1/2 Cup of Gluten Free Oatmeal

1 Cup of Almond Milk

1/4 Cup of Almonds

1/2 Cup of Berries

1 tsp of Ground Cinnamon

NUTRITIONAL VALUE

Fat: 21 g/ Carbs: 40 g/ Protein: 12 g

Total Calories: 401 Calories

DIRECTIONS

In a pot place the oats, cinnamon and the almond milk and turn the heat on high until it starts boiling. Once it's boiling turn the heat down to low and stir until all of the almond milk is absorbed. Once the oatmeal is ready transfer it into a bowl and add the nuts and fresh berries.

Optional: Add honey or extra toppings.

CHOCOLATE OVERNIGHT OATS

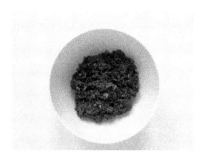

INGREDIENTS

1/2 Cup of Gluten Free Oatmeal

1 Cup of Almond Milk

1 Serving of Chocolate Protein Powder

1 Tbsp of Chia Seeds

1 Tbsp of Raw Cacao Powder

1 Tbsp of Maple Syrup

Optional: Raw Cacao Nibs

NUTRITIONAL VALUE

Fat: 18 g/ Carbs: 60 g/ Protein: 46 g

Total Calories: 550 Calories

DIRECTIONS

Combine all the ingredients into a mason jar or a sealed container, give it a good stir and place in the fridge overnight. In the morning, add raw cacao nibs on top for an extra crunch if desired. Enjoy cold or heated up.

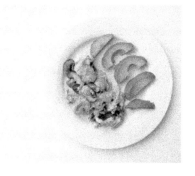

INGREDIENTS

2 Eggs

1 Cup of Spinach

2 Mushrooms

1/4 Red Bell Pepper

1/4 Cup of Red Onions

1/2 Avocado

1 tsp of Coconut Oil

NUTRITIONAL VALUE

Fat: 39 g/ Carbs: 16 g/ Protein: 16 g

Total Calories: 460 Calories

DIRECTIONS

Heat a pan on medium heat and add the coconut oil. Once the coconut oil is melted add all of the vegetables except for the spinach and cook for 3 minutes. Finally add the eggs and spinach. Once the omelette is complete add the sliced avocado on top. Season with salt and pepper to your desire.

MINI OMELETTES

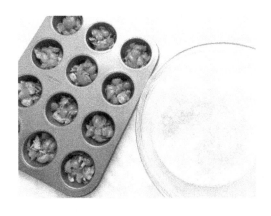

INGREDIENTS

3 Eggs

1/2 Cup of Spinach

1 Small Tomato

1 Tbsp of Fresh Basil

1 Tbsp of Coconut Oil

NUTRITIONAL VALUE

Fat: 29 g/ Carbs: 5 g/ Protein: 20 g

Total Calories: 360 Calories

DIRECTIONS

Preheat the oven at 350F/175C. Coat a muffin tray with coconut oil to avoid sticking. Whisk together the 3 eggs. Chop up the spinach, basil and tomatoes. Pour the egg mixture into 3 different muffin cups. Then add a little bit of the vegetable mixture in each cup leaving about 1cm empty at the top. Bake in the oven for 18 minutes.

BANANA PANCAKES

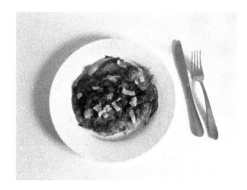

INGREDIENTS

1 Banana

2 Eggs

1 tsp of Ground Cinnamon

1 tsp of Coconut Oil

NUTRITIONAL VALUE

Fat: 24 g/ Carbs: 30 g/ Protein: 14 g

Total Calories: 378 Calories

DIRECTIONS

In a bowl combine the banana and two eggs. Use a hand blender or a fork to mix the banana and eggs together. You should end up with a consistency similar to pancake batter. Place a pan on medium heat and melt the coconut oil. Slowly add the batter in the pan forming 5-inch diameter pancakes. Put the cover on and cook for 30 seconds on each side. Repeat until you have cooked the whole batch. Be creative with your toppings, add any of your favorite clean foods. These may include but are not limited to berries, almond butter, coconut flakes and chopped nuts.

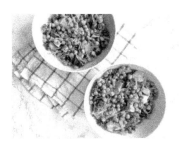

INGREDIENTS

2 Cups of Kale/ 1 Carrot

1/2 Avocado1/2 Cup of Chickpeas

Dressing —>

1 Tbsp of Tahini

1 Tbsp of Lemon Juice

NUTRITIONAL VALUE

Fat: 22 g/ Carbs: 40 g/ Protein: 16 g

Total Calories: 431 Calories

DIRECTIONS

Preheat the oven to 350F/175C. Drain and rinse the chickpeas. Dry them with a paper towel and spread them evenly on a baking tray. Bake for 45 minutes. While the chickpeas are baking prepare the vegetables by rinsing and chopping up the kale, peeling and shredding the carrots and cutting the avocado into small cubes. Set the vegetables aside and prepare the dressing. Combine all the dressing ingredients into a bowl and whisk together until it forms a smooth consistency. Add all of the vegetables to a bowl with the baked chickpeas and then drizzle the dressing on top.

TUNA WRAP

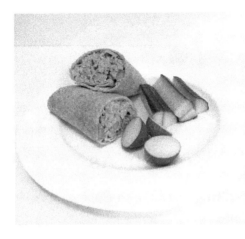

INGREDIENTS

1 Can of Tuna

1/2 Avocado

2 Stalks of Celery

1/4 Cup of Red Onions

2 Brown Rice Tortilla Wraps

NUTRITIONAL VALUE

Fat: 17 g/ Carbs: 43 g/ Protein: 38 g

Total Calories: 453 Calories

DIRECTIONS

Drain the can of tuna and pour it into a mixing bowl. Scoop out half of an avocado and mix it in with the tuna. Finely chop the celery and red onion and add to the bowl. Season with salt and pepper. Add the mixture to the brown rice tortilla wraps and roll.

SWEET POTATO SALMON CAKES

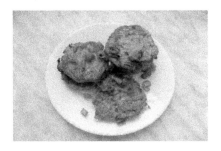

INGREDIENTS

(2 Servings)

1 Medium Sweet Potato/ 8 oz Salmon Filet

1 Egg/ 1/2 Cup of Almond Flour

1/4 Cup of Green Onions/ 1 tsp of Sea Salt

1/4 tsp of Black Pepper

NUTRITIONAL VALUE

(per serving)

Fat: 25 g/ Carbs: 25 g/ Protein: 30 g

Total Calories: 434 Calories

DIRECTIONS

Preheat the oven at 400F/200C and line a baking sheet with parchment paper. Wash and peel the sweet potato and steam until soft. Bake the salmon for about 15-20 minutes. Once the sweet potato is soft and the salmon is cooked mash them up in a bowl and add in the remaining ingredients. Form 8 patties and spread them out on the baking sheet. Bake the Sweet Potato Salmon cakes for 30 minutes, flip the patties at around 15 minutes. Serve it on its own or with a green salad.

ZUCCHINI NOODLES & BOLOGNESE

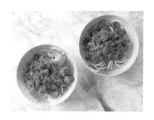

INGREDIENTS

(2 Servings) 2 Zucchinis

450 g of Ground Beef/ 1/2 Cup of Coconut Milk

1/4 Cup of Tomato Paste/ 1 Cup of Spinach/ 1 Carrot/ 6 Mushrooms

1/2 Cup of Onions/ 2 Cloves of Garlic/ 1 Tbsp of Coconut Oil

NUTRITIONAL VALUE

(per serving)

Fat: 25 g/ Carbs: 10 g/ Protein: 28 g

Total Calories: 374 Calories

DIRECTIONS

Chop the onions, garlic and mushrooms. In a pan melt the coconut oil and add the onions and garlic, once the onions become translucent add in the ground beef and season with salt and pepper. Once the ground beef is cooked through, add the chopped mushrooms and spinach. In a small bowl combine the coconut milk and tomato paste and mix together until it forms a thick sauce. Add the coconut milk and tomato paste mixture to the skillet and turn the heat down to low, let simmer for about 10 minutes. While the Bolognese is cooking wash 1 zucchini and spiralize it into noodles. Serve the Bolognese on top of the spiralized zucchini.

The fact that you reached this level in the book shows the commitment you took to make that change for your body and Health. This is why I love sharing the knowledge I have and this is what keeps me motivated to learn more. For that reason, I will share with you more than 20 clean eating recipes, 4 Weeks eating plan, and the grocery list needed as a FREE BONUS.

Visit **http://bit.ly/2FyBVMR** to get your BONUS of 20 clean eating recipes, 4 Weeks eating plan, and the grocery list needed

Eating out while on a healthy eating lifestyle

Committing to a clean eating lifestyle doesn't mean you will never be able to attend social events or dine out again. When you switch to a clean eating lifestyle you have to make sure that it fits into your lifestyle. Although going out every night of the week is not recommended, going out once in a while will be healthy for you if it's something you really enjoy.

It's a matter of making the right choices. Look for dishes like stir-fries and salads on the menu. If you can't find anything on the menu that is clean eating approved here are some examples of things you can order separately

Protein
Grilled Chicken Breast
Grilled Salmon Fillet
Steak
Hamburger without the bun

Carbs
Baked Potato
Baked Sweet Potato Fries
Quinoa
Brown Rice

Fats
Avocado or Guacamole
Nuts and Seeds (Great on salads)
Olive Oil

Beverages
Water
Sparkling Water
Tea
Coffee

Most of the restaurants will have all of these foods in the kitchen even if it's not written exactly like that on the menu. Don't be shy to ask for something a little different. When it comes to your health it's always worth it. The last tip for eating out on a clean eating diet is to ALWAYS ask for the dressing on the side. Most restaurants add way more than needed. Even if it's a healthy dressing I recommend doing this.

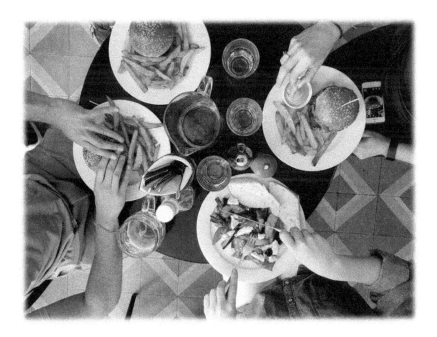

Chapter 4: Intermittent Fasting

Exercises

Exercises will help to increase the fat burning process of the body when combined with intermittent fasting. And for those who are interested in building or maintaining muscles mass, exercise during fasting is a great way to achieve that.

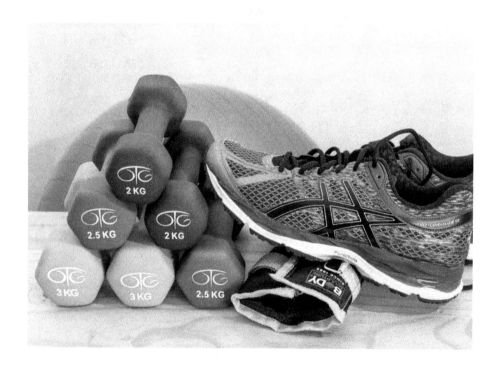

Benefits of Exercising in a Fasted State

Studies have shown that exercising in a fasted state is capable of significantly decreasing levels of body fat and weight (Mercola, 2013, n.p.).

There are studies that show that exercising in a fasted state can lead to acute oxidative stress. Working out during fasting is likely to slow down the aging process of your muscles and rejuvenate your brain cells. To put it simply: exercising during fasting is capable of keeping your brain cells and muscle tissues young. (Mercola, 2011, n.p.).

In addition to the above, some other benefits include:

- A significant increase in the production of growth hormones.

- Increased chances of slowing down depression.

- It perks up the resilience, elasticity, and flexibility of muscles.

Workouts according to goals

Now, I'm well aware that each and every one of you reading this, has individual characteristics and different goals, which is exactly why, I'm giving you a 4 days per week workout, that will target all of the 3 goals below-

1. Strength gaining
2. Muscle building (looking better)
3. Fat loss

The importance of resistance training during fat loss

As you may or may not know, when subjected to a caloric deficit, the body burns both fat and muscle tissue. The bigger the deficit, the more you lose of both and last but not least, the more your metabolism slows down.

We can look at fat tissue as an energy reserve, using which, the body compensates for the deficit of energy from food (and hence, losing fat/weight).

That fat tissue is an inactive tissue, meaning it cannot do any work. On the flipside, however, we have the ACTIVE tissue, which the muscles are.

It is of PRIME IMPORTANCE to train your muscles during a period of weight loss, whether you are a man or a woman.

Engaging your muscles while on a deficit will GREATLY help you MAINTAIN that muscle tissue. That in turn, will keep your metabolism higher. Why? Because muscles require more energy (food) to be maintained and can do more work (burn calories).

So, if you lose your muscle tissue, your body literally says "I don't need that much food" and the TDEE increases. (Walker, Cheryl, and Alicia Roberts, 2017)

Bottom line is that having more muscle mass helps you burn more calories even at rest and furthermore, helps you burn more during activity. So, why wouldn't you train your muscles?

Before I move into the workouts, I will briefly explain to you a bit more about the musculature of the human body, how it works and how it adapts. All of this is important, simply because, working with a machine becomes easier and more intuitive, when you know its functions and separate parts.

In that case, the machine is the body and the separate functional parts are the muscles.

Muscle growth

As I said earlier in the benefits section, gaining muscle is a direct function of exercising, but what do I mean by that?

We can simply look at muscle gaining as to a type of adaptation. A positive adaptation for that matter.

In order for the body to increase its muscle mass, we MUST subject it to previously unexperienced stress. Of course, that previously unexperienced stress (overload), combined with proper recovery windows and nutrition, leads to that type of positive adaptation. (Hernandez, Kravitz, 2003)

Is all muscle growth the same?

Well, some people associate muscle gains with strength gains. While this statement is logically true, being at your strongest doesn't mean you will be at your biggest size and vice versa.

In other words, there are different types of hypertrophy (the scientific term for growth). So, let us take a closer look at them and see what function each type of growth has. After that, later on in the book, I'm going to show you a couple of workouts for different types of goals (strength gains, bulk muscle gains, fat loss).

Types of muscle growth

There are two types of muscle hypertrophy- Myofibril hypertrophy and Sarcoplasmic hypertrophy

The myofibrils are the contractile elements of the muscles, which we refer to as "muscle fibers", in simple terms. Hence, **myofibril hypertrophy** is an increase in the size of these muscle fibers.

This type of muscle growth is mostly sought by strength athletes, such as powerlifters, strongmen and Olympic weight lifters. Why? Because myofibril hypertrophy results directly in increased strength levels, or in other words- Relative strength.

This is simply, strength, referred to the body weight of the individual. In other words, myofibril hypertrophy doesn't lead to a significant increase in weight and muscle bulk, but rather a stronger musculature. Bottom line is that myofibril hypertrophy serves as means of increasing maximum strength capabilities, rather than maximum muscle bulk.

On the other hand, we have **sarcoplasmic hypertrophy.** While the myofibrils are the muscle fibers, the sarcoplasm is that jelly-like fluid surrounding those muscle fibers. The fluid is made up of non-contractile proteins, energy substances and water.

The increase in volume of that sarcoplasm, we refer to as "Sarcoplasmic hypertrophy". That type of muscle growth is essentially a function of an increased training volume.

The main end results we achieve with sarcoplasmic hypertrophy are namely the "bulk muscle gains", which is why this type of hypertrophy is mostly looked for by physique athletes, whose main goals are being at their biggest, leanest, most symmetrical and aesthetic shapes.

Needless to say, sarcoplasmic hypertrophy also leads to strength gains, but those strength gains are not as prominent as with myofibril hypertrophy, which is exactly why they are just an accompanying aspect.

Why is all that important?

As I already mentioned, it is of prime importance to understand how the body reacts to the stimulus you're giving it. In other words, you have to know what you are doing, before you start doing it.

So, let's recap here- Being at your strongest doesn't really mean being at your biggest and vice versa. That is simply due to the different types of adaptations the musculature goes through.

The type of adaptation depends on the type of training, so let's start off by giving you two separate workouts.

The workout

The training will be oriented towards **INTENSITY.** If you happen to be unaware of that, intensity is a characteristic of the workload, that defines how close we get to our maximum strength capabilities.

Note- Compound movements engage more than 1 joint and muscle group.

What we have is a strength & cardio.. Wait, what? Well, I am serious, you can build muscle and strength while building a better cardiorespiratory system. And I am not just referring to the cardiovascular benefits of usual, steady state cardio, that accounts for a better blood feeding of the musculature.

	Name		Date	
	Metabolic Chaos		Wk 1- Day 1	

Order	Range of Motion, Activation, Movement Prep	Sets	Reps	Work	Rest	Notes:
	Foam Roll Series	1				
	Lat Band Walk	1	15e			
	Glute Bridge w/ Band	1	20			
	SL Glute Bridge	1	10e			
	Floor Sliders	1	15			
	Shoulder Flexion	1	15			
	Yoga Pushup	1	15			
	Gate Swings	2	15			

Order	Movement	Exercise	Sets	Reps	Work	Rest	Notes:
A1	Power	KB DLHP	1		20 sec	10 sec	**1-2 Minute Rest b/t rounds**
B1	Energy System	Mountain Climbers	1		20 sec	10 sec	-Switch sides for split squat
C1	Core	Knee grabs	1		20 sec	10 sec	every other round (L,R,L,R)
D1	Quad	DB Split Squat	1		20 sec	10 sec	
E1	Pull	BB Inverted Row *Underhand*	1		20 sec	10 sec	
F1	Hip	KB Deadlift	1		20 sec	10 sec	
G1	Press	DB Floor Press	1		20 sec	10 sec	
H1	Core	Sitouts	1		20 sec	10 sec	

# of rounds	6 Rounds

Order	Finisher	Sets	Reps	Work	Rest	Notes:
						Omit

Visit: http://bit.ly/workoutstrainics

to get your BONUS of daily WODs of 6 months

Pre- and Post-Workout Fasting

Having seen the types of exercises as well as the benefits of performing them during fasting, the likely question is if you should exercise before or during your fasting window. In other words, when is the best time to exercise – just before you break your fast, right after breaking your fast, in the middle of your eating window, or in the middle of your fasting window?

Here's a short answer: all are just fine.

And here's the long answer.

Working out in a fasted state increases your body's ability to burn fat. There are studies which show that when you eat before you workout, your blood sugar increases both before and during the workout. (Scandinavian Journal of Medicine and Science in Sports, 2018, n.p.), (Gleeson, M. et al. 1986, 55: 645). This makes perfect sense, especially if your meal before the exercise contains sufficient amounts of carbohydrates.

Exercising in a fasted state means that your body gets its energy from the breakdown of body fat. Another study of 273 subjects shows that burning of fat was significantly higher while exercising in a fasted state. However, in a fed state, insulin and glucose levels were significantly higher (The British Journal of Nutrition, 2016, n.p.).

All these metabolic activities involving either the usage of carbohydrates or fat shows that your body can function perfectly well with or without the recent intake of food (American Journal of Psychology, Endocrinology and Metabolism, 2012, n.p.).

Do What's Convenient and Healthy for You

Exercising in the mornings while fasting may be a great idea but it usually leaves you dealing with post-workout hunger. However, if this is a non-issue for you, there's no harm in exercising in the mornings before going about your day's activities. This simply means that if you wake up around 6 am and do your exercises for about an hour, you are going to wait for between 6 to 8 hours (depending on your fasting window) before your first meal.

Scheduling your fast in the afternoons may be ideal timing but it is difficult to fit that into a busy day's schedule for most people. Eating between 1 to 2 hours after your workout session is a great way to allow your body to recover from the stress of exercising. This, however, means that if your fasting window ends by 2 pm, for example, you will have to start exercising around 1 pm. This is not feasible for most people especially those who have a 9 to 5 job.

Perhaps moving the workout to evenings will be best. But there are those who think that exercising in the evening may interfere with their body rhythms and sleep patterns leading to insomnia.

This all comes down to personal preference. There is no one-size-fits-all when it comes to combining fasting and exercise. Find what suits or works for your health and schedule and remember to stay well hydrated while combining fasting with exercises.

Does Exercising in a Fasted State Burn Muscle?

The fear for many people who want to build or maintain lean muscle is that they will eventually lose muscle if they exercise on an empty stomach because, in the absence of food, muscle tissues will be broken down and converted to glucose to fuel the body during exercise.

According to Dr. Fung, the body does not use muscle tissues as fuel when we exercise in a fasted state. While it is possible to not gain or build muscle by exercising in a fasted state, the body only burns fat and not muscle when you exercise whether in a fasted or fed state. He further argues that if our bodies are intelligent enough to store up fat so that it can be used when there is no supply of glucose, it is also intelligent enough not to use muscle tissues as an alternative source of energy in the absence of food. In his words, *"Protein is functional tissue and has many purposes other than energy storage, whereas fat is specialized for energy storage. Would it not make sense that you would use fat for energy instead of protein? That is kind of like storing firewood for heat. But as soon as you need heat, you chop up your sofa and throw it into the fire. That is completely idiotic and that is not the way our bodies are designed to work"* (Fung, 2017, n.p.).

Here is a study that shows our muscle mass is intact even when we exercise in a fasted state. The US National Library of Medicine published a study titled, *"The Protein-retaining Effects of Growth Hormone during Fasting Involve Inhibition of Muscle-protein Breakdown"* (US National Library of Medicine, 2011, n.p.) which reveals that growth hormones are actually responsible for keeping muscle mass intact during fasting.

The study administered a drug that inhibited the production of growth hormones in subjects while they were made to fast. Interestingly, there was about a 50% increase in the breakdown of their muscles simply by suppressing their growth hormones. This is a strong indication that growth hormones play an important role in maintaining lean muscles.

Chapter 5: Intermittent Fasting for Men versus Women

Fasting may be considered a very good and healthy practice for most people. However, there is a growing concern about the effect it has on the different sexes. The way the male body tolerates long periods of absence of food is quite different from the way the female body does. While male hormones may have a strong tolerance for fasting, the female's cortisol, progesterone, insulin, leptin, and estrogen may go completely out of order if their natural rhythm or balance is interfered with by long absence of food.

Here are some of the impacts of fasting on hormones. Note that these impacts may not be the same for everyone.

Effect on Hormonal Balance

Our numerous hormones are designed to be at equilibrium for our bodies to function optimally. But when stress is introduced in the body, it begins to cause an imbalance in hormone levels. Cortisol, the stress hormone, is released by the adrenal gland to regulate stress. Fasting is known to affect the functioning of cortisol in some women. This means, in some women, going without food for longer periods than their body is used to may keep their cortisol level constantly high or constantly low. Or it might keep the cortisol level low when it should be high and high when it should be low.

Another hormone that is likely to be affected by intermittent fasting are the thyroid hormones. In both male and females, the thyroid hormone affects every single cell in the body. This is why if you have a history of thyroid disorder you should seek expert advice before commencing intermittent fasting.

Effect on Reproductive Hormones

The male and female bodies are different and thus, react differently to changes in eating habits or patterns. The reason for this difference in the way both sexes react to fasting may not be too certain, but studies have suggested that it may be connected to the protein molecule which is responsible for transmitting messages between neurons. This protein molecule is known as kisspeptin. The function of kisspeptin in men is the production of testosterone which is responsible for reproduction. In women, kisspeptin boosts the production of estrogen and progesterone – the hormones responsible for ovulation.

The reproductive hormones in both males and females are interconnected to other hormones such as leptin, ghrelin, and insulin – all of which are responsible for triggering feelings of hunger and satiation. In women, however, the level of kisspeptin is higher than in men, therefore, their bodies are more sensitive to the slightest hormonal imbalance. This tends to affect their overall body energy balance. This may explain why when women go without food for longer periods than their bodies are used to, their kisspeptin levels decrease sharply and this could affect their reproductive hormones.

While there may not be any available studies to show the effect of fasting on female reproductive hormones, there are, however, studies that show the results of fasting on female rats. This means, for now, science has not provided any concrete evidence using human females, therefore, caution is required for females who want to practice intermittent fasting.

What does this mean for women who want to practice intermittent fasting? Should women avoid fasting altogether? Will intermittent fasting ruin the chances for women to get pregnant? Is intermittent fasting recommended only for women who have gone past the reproductive age?

This all comes down to individual differences. There is no one particular hard and fast rule for every woman (and even men for that matter) when it comes to intermittent fasting. With all the different anecdotal accounts from different women – some fervently supporting and some vehemently opposing intermittent fasting, it is difficult to say what is right for every woman. It is only safe to say that every woman should proceed with the understanding that their bodies are unique. This is why it is very necessary to seek the advice of a medical expert especially when the woman is unsure of her suitability for the practice or if there has been any history of health challenges.

Effect on Autophagy

While it is true that intermittent fasting can activate autophagy especially in men, this may not necessarily be true for women.

A study conducted in this regard indicates that male neurons react to fasting by activating autophagy but female neurons react to fasting by hampering autophagy. According to the study, *"The role of autophagy during starvation is both sex- and tissue-dependent."* During starvation, neurons from males more readily undergo autophagy and die, whereas neurons from females mobilize fatty acids, accumulate triglycerides, form lipid droplets, and survive longer. (US National Library of Medicine, 2009, n.p.).

This does not translate to mean that autophagy is not achievable for women. It only takes more time for women to get into a state of autophagy than men. The *Journal of Cardiovascular Translational Research* pointed out that having some level of resistance to autophagy may actually be an advantage as some diseases can piggyback on autophagy to cause havoc to the human body. This makes women less vulnerable to these diseases (Journal of Cardiovascular Translational Research, 2014, p.182-191).

The Positive Effect of Perceptions

One underlying factor in the way fasting affects both the male and female body is our perception. If we perceive fasting as stress activating activity, then our bodies must react negatively to it. There may not be any hard evidence of the role of our perceptions on how they affect intermittent fasting, but there is no denying the fact that our bodies react to our overall state of mind. Considering evidence like the placebo effect and how the body reacts to dreams or nightmares, we can only agree that our minds and bodies cannot differentiate between a perceived or real event.

Considering the above, intermittent fasting is not a practice you should take up based solely on inspiration. Being pragmatic is vital when our health is on the line.

Are Men More Suitable for Fasting than Women?

Following that logic and train of thought, the question of whether or not fasting is suitable for women still remains. There are TONS of articles on this topic, as well as many women who claimed that their health declined, due to fasting.

Excessive stress of any kind can signal the body to quite literally, turn off secondary functions and systems like the reproductive system.

Many people, both men and women, report negative effects upon their health, due to a newly started training or nutrition regimen. And that's not only because of the badly structured regimen, but also, because of the means of application of the end user.

That is to say that people have a tendency to take everything to the extremes, without ever finding the proper balance. A badly structured regimen, followed up with an exorbitant approach, logically leads to a negative impact on the body.

For example- We either do ZERO physical activity or we beat our bodies. We either eat too much or too little, with the latter one being in an expectation to lose weight.

Now, many of the people who report negative side effects due to fasting, claim it is dangerous because it subjects the body to caloric restrictions.

But is that the main factor, making that statement a hundred percent correct and disproving all of fasting's benefits? I don't think so.

As a matter of fact, fasting is not just recommended for weight loss (a caloric deficit). You can also do it in a muscle building period, with no worries. It's all about food distribution, quantity and quality, both during weight loss and muscle gain.

If you think fasting can damage your body, well, 16 hours with no food is really not all that much. The body has its own reserves, which allow us to last without food for quite a bit of time, before we experience negative outcomes.

Of course, during that time when the body is deprived of food, we have to take in account other factors, in order to remain mentally sharp and physically energetic.

So, we have to provide our bodies with a good amount of water and other liquids like tea, all while avoiding toxic habits like drinking alcohol.

Not only does fasting not have negative outcomes, if done properly, but the short-term, micro stress it imposes the body to is actually beneficial and leads to positive adaptations.

The important and key words here are "short-term and micro", as prolonged, big stress is really not beneficial. In big quantities, cure is poison and vice versa.

Specifically, for fasting & females, one of women's problems with IF arise from the facts that when paying attention to their nutrition, they overthink the word "restriction". Women tend to significantly restrict themselves of energy (food), restrict the diversity of their food sources and that way, they reach the extremes, where they don't give their body enough of what it needs to sustain a healthy, properly functioning inner environment.

If you calculate your intake, acknowledge the benefits and have a solid dinner as a last meal of your time window during IF.. Well, there is absolutely no reason for the body to not last without food, healthily, until your next eating window starts.

If, however, you're a female that is literally afraid of her food and barely consumes 100 calories at the last meal, then the next 16 hours would be a nightmare for the body.

Furthermore, if you add a workout during the fasting window, the body will quite literally panic and negative outcomes will be the end result.

Females' issues with intermittent fasting- Summed up

There may be no scientific evidence to show that men are more suitable to fast than women. However, anything that is capable of destabilizing a woman's reproductive system is also capable of throwing her overall health out of balance. So, whether you are a woman in the reproductive age or not, caution is required when practicing intermittent fasting. A woman who notices the following should pause fasting and seek for medical advice:

- Complete stoppage or increased irregularity in menstrual cycle

- Longer periods for injuries to heal

- Longer periods to fully recover from workouts

- Catching common bugs easily

- Increased rate in the frequency of mood swings

- A significant decline in the ability to tolerate stress

- A significant decline in food digestion time

- Feeling cold most of the time even when you are not ill

- Hair beginning to fall off

- Increase in skin dryness

- Increased appearance of acne

- Having difficulty falling asleep or any issue with insomnia

- Increased irregularity in heartbeats

Challenges with Intermittent Fasting

A simple Google search about intermittent fasting will reveal many results about the many excellent benefits of intermittent fasting. It is not surprising as many scientific studies trumpet the praise of intermittent fasting. A certain study affirmed that intermittent fasting alongside calorie restriction helps improve cardiovascular health and helped obese women lose weight (University of Adelaide, 2019, n.p)

However, as studies are revealing the praises of intermittent fasting, some come as a warning as well.

All in all, there are some challenges that people should watch out for when practicing intermittent fasting.

The Possibility of an Unhealthy Obsession with Food

You have stayed away from food all morning, and you suddenly see your partner eating. All that occupies your mind is what you will eat when breaking your fast at dinner.

Hunger has been a reliable mechanism that keeps man alive. With the availability of grocery stores, restaurants, and fast food everywhere, hunger hardly becomes a problem. However, the problem comes when you are fasting as you tend to be obsessed with planning your meal.

Everything becomes about food.

Possibility of Inflammation and Food Intolerance

Fasting leaves you hungry, creating the likelihood of succumbing to anything you find edible. Many people, in their bid to soothe their cravings, overload on calories. They resort to food high in dairy, gluten, and other reactive food in excess. This could trigger leaky gut, food intolerance, as well as inflammation

According to a study in the Immunology Journal, when mice were fed with gluten, they suffered from inflammation, increasing their risk for Type 1 diabetes. Inflammation has been a significant contributor to weight gain. (Julie C Antvorskov *et al*, 2012). For this reason, you have to follow the steps to know how to break your fasts and avoid this possible challenge.

Blood Sugar Levels have to be maintained

The blood sugar level of the body is so vital that it shouldn't be too high or too low. Eating healthy and regularly really does help to keep the body's glycemic index stable. During fasting, however, the reverse happens.

Intermittent fasting can trigger a hypoglycemic state (low blood sugar levels) in the body (Laura, C. 2018. n.p). This will disturb the delicate balance of blood sugar levels in the body. This is one of the challenges of intermittent fasting which could cause excessive weakness and abnormal drowsiness for certain people. (Mohammad Alsaggar, 2016).

A Tendency to Over-Depend on Coffee

While practicing intermittent fasting, you can use coffee to suppress hunger pangs. Hence, many people find themselves gulping cups after cups of coffee to keep them going. The negative side, however, is that excessive caffeine could affect your sleep cycle.

"It is a vicious cycle, as caffeine can disrupt sleep and promotes anxiety and depression," writes Mark Hyman, M.D. (Mark Hyman, MD, 2012).

In addition, coffee also raises cortisol levels (stress hormones). Cortisol raises the blood glucose level. This can increase blood sugar levels and raise insulin resistance as well.

Intermittent Fasting Tips and Hacks

Intermittent fasting doesn't have to be a punishment or a lifestyle that will make your life difficult. Yes, going without food could be uncomfortable, but it is not impossible. Over the years, experts have developed tricks to make intermittent fasting easy and help people reap immense benefits with the lifestyle.

A few intermittent fasting tips and hacks include:

Add Brain Octane Oil to your meals

A high-quality MCT oil such as Brain Octane Oil in your food will fast track the benefits of intermittent fasting. Therefore, you enjoy maximum weight loss while suppressing hunger pangs. Additionally, Brain Octane creates ketones in the body.

Concentrate on Healthy Meals

Many people feel they can reward themselves with whatever they want after hours of fasting. This is a bad idea; instead, focus on healthy, balanced, and whole foods that ensure you get the vital nutrients. With this, your hormones stabilize and you have optimal energy levels while fasting.

Stay Away from Artificially Flavored Drinks

Fasting is not the time to drink diet soda, fruit juice, flavored beverages, and other energy drinks even if they claim to be low in sugar. Even without sugar, they are laden with artificial sweeteners and additives. Some of them use addictive like Sweet & Low which tend to make you overeat.

Drink More Water

Most of the time, the body interprets dehydration as a sign of hunger. This is why it is essential to drink enough water while fasting. Even while eating, ensure to drink adequate water. Water has the tendency of keeping you full, which can prevent overeating.

To spice things up, try and include herbs and fresh fruits. This is detoxifying, healthy, and tasty.

Pick a Conducive Time Frame

One of the best parts of intermittent fasting is flexibility. There is no strict rule you have to follow in terms of time. Intermittent fasting has many techniques that you can adapt to suit your lifestyle. Either the 20:4 method, the 16: 8 approach, OMAD, etc, you can choose when you want to start based on your schedule. If you don't like skipping breakfast, for instance, you could schedule your fast from 11 am to 5 pm, if you prefer the 16:8 method.

Part of the reason some people fail with intermittent fasting is that they restrict themselves to someone else's schedule. However, intermittent fasting is personal, and it is a lifestyle; hence, you need to plan out the fast carefully, so you don't exhaust yourself.

Be sure to be creative with choosing your fasting time. Try and schedule the majority of your fasting period to your sleep period.

Conclusion

The same way you treat your skin and nails to a spa treatment, intermittent fasting is also a spa for the whole body. With intermittent fasting, you flush toxins from the entire body and avail your body system of the opportunity to heal itself and to take in high-quality nutrients. You give your body organs, cells, and tissues some relaxation time while your body burns fat.

There are many benefits of intermittent fasting; I will, however, recommend you to approach it from a neutral perspective. If you are after weight loss, be sure to follow the steps provided – watch your calorie and macronutrient intake.

While intermittent fasting works without a doubt, you have to play your part. Stay away from processed foods, junk food, and sugar-laden foods. Be sure to focus solely on a balanced diet, drink enough water during your fast to suppress hunger pangs.

I love intermittent fasting in that it differs from many weight loss diets out there. It doesn't come with many health restrictions that many weight loss diet places on users. You get to eat what you want within the healthy food realm and enjoy tremendous health benefits. Rather than common diets that constrict you and make life uncomfortable, intermittent fasting is a lifestyle. You grow and make the needed commitment to reap the benefits.

On a final note, be sure to listen to your body to determine the fast that works best for you. People differ in terms of age, activity level, level of body fat, and how healthy they are. As a result, what works for one might not work for the other. Listen to your body, progress gradually and grow into it.

Thank you again for reading this book!

I hope it was able to help you discover the Intermittent fasting lifestyle and its benefits.

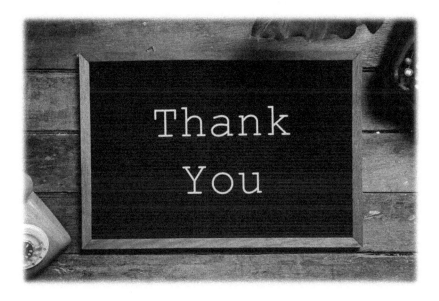

Finally, if you enjoyed this book, then I'd like to ask you for a favor, would you be kind enough to leave a review for this book on Amazon? It'd be greatly appreciated!

Thank you and good luck!

Let's upgrade our bodies

References

American Journal of Managed Care. (2013). *Targeting insulin resistance: The ongoing paradigm shift in diabetes prevention.* Retrieved from http://www.ajmc.com/journals/evidence-based-diabetes-management/2013/2013-1-vol19-sp2/targeting-insulin-resistance-the-ongoing-paradigm-shift-in-diabetes-prevention

American Journal of Psychology, Endocrinology and Metabolism. (2012). *Adaptive reciprocity of lipid and glucose metabolism in human short-term starvation.* Retrieved from https://www.ncbi.nlm.nih.gov/pubmed/23074240

Antunes, Fernanda, et al. "Autophagy and Intermittent Fasting: the Connection for Cancer Therapy?" *Clinics (Sao Paulo, Brazil)*, Hospital Das Clínicas Da Faculdade De Medicina Da Universidade De São Paulo, 27 Nov. 2018, www.ncbi.nlm.nih.gov/pmc/articles/PMC6257056/.

Arlene, S. (2016) *Post-Workout Nutrition: What to Eat After a Workout.* Retrieved from https://www.healthline.com/nutrition/eat-after-workout/

Berg, E. (2019). *Overcoming Adrenal Stress with Intermittent Fasting.* Retrieved from https://www.drberg.com/blog/overcoming-adrenal-stress-with-intermittent-fasting

Body and Soul, (2016). *What do sugar cravings mean?* Retrieved from https://www.bodyandsoul.com.au/health/health-news/what-do-sugar-cravings-mean/news-story/ccbe0aac221ecb8c9768add7a9bccefd

Catterson, James H et al. "Short-Term, Intermittent Fasting Induces Long-Lasting Gut Health and TOR-Independent Lifespan Extension" *Current biology : CB* vol. 28,11 (2018): 1714-1724.e4.

Cleveland Clinic, (2013) *Fat and Calories*. Retrieved from https://my.clevelandclinic.org/health/articles/4182-fat-and-calories/

Dorff, Tanya B, et al. "Safety and Feasibility of Fasting in Combination with Platinum-Based Chemotherapy." *BMC Cancer*, BioMed Central, 10 June 2016, www.ncbi.nlm.nih.gov/pmc/articles/PMC4901417/.

Dr. Vedrana, H. (2018). *Intermittent fasting, your thyroid, and your immune system.* Retrieved from https://medium.com/boosted/intermittent-fasting-your-thyroid-and-your-immune-system-ec8f5f02d997

Fung, J. (2016). *How does fasting affect your brain?* Retrieved from https://www.dietdoctor.com/fasting-affect-brain/

Fung, J. (2017). *Fasting and muscle mass*. Retrieved from https://www.dietdoctor.com/fasting-muscle-mass

Fung, J. (2018). *Fasting and Muscle Mass – Fasting Part 15.* Retrieved from https://idmprogram.com/fasting-and-muscle-mass-fasting-part-14/

Gleeson, M., Maughan, R.J. & Greenhaff, P.L. Europ. J. Appl. Physiol. (1986) 55: 645. *Comparison of the effects of pre-exercise feeding of glucose, glycerol and placebo on endurance and fuel homeostasis in man.* Retrieved from https://doi.org/10.1007/BF00423211

Gotthardt, Juliet D et al. "Intermittent Fasting Promotes Fat Loss With Lean Mass Retention, Increased

Hypothalamic Norepinephrine Content, and Increased Neuropeptide Y Gene Expression in Diet-Induced Obese Male Mice"*Endocrinology* vol. 157,2 (2015): 679-91.

Harvard Health Publishing. "Obesity: Unhealthy and Unmanly." *Harvard Health*, Mar. 2011, www.health.harvard.edu/mens-health/obesity-unhealthy-and-unmanly.

Hernandez, Richard Joshua, and Len Kravitz. "The Mystery of Skeletal Muscle Hypertrophy." *Skeletal Muscle Hypertrophy*, ACSM'S Health & Fitness Journal, 2003, www.unm.edu/~lkravitz/Article folder/hypertrophy.html.

Ho, K Y et al. "Fasting enhances growth hormone secretion and amplifies the complex rhythms of growth hormone secretion in man" *Journal of clinical investigation* vol. 81,4 (1988): 968-75.

Journal of Cardiovascular Translational Research. (2014). *The role of sex differences in autophagy in the heart during coxsackievirus b3-induced myocarditis.* Retrieved from https://link.springer.com/article/10.1007/s12265-013-9525-5

Julie, C. (2012). *Dietary gluten alters the balance of pro-inflammatory and anti-inflammatory cytokines in T cells of BALB/c mice.* Retrieved from https://www.ncbi.nlm.nih.gov/pmc/articles/PMC3533698/

Katy, A. (2018). *Study links processed carb consumption to weight gain.* Retrieved from https://www.foodnavigator.com/Article/2018/01/03/Study-links-processed-carb-consumption-to-weight-gain/

Kollias, H. (2018). *Intermittent fasting for women: Important information you need to know.* Retrieved from https://www.precisionnutrition.com/intermittent-fasting-women

Krista, A. *et al.* (2007). *Alternate-day fasting and chronic disease prevention: a review of human and animal trials.* Retrieved from https://academic.oup.com/ajcn/article/86/1/7/4633143

Kumar S., Kaur, G. (2013). *Intermittent fasting dietary restriction regimen negatively influences reproduction in young rats: A study of hypothalamo-hypophysial-gonadal axis.* Retrieved from PLoS ONE 8(1): e52416. https://doi.org/10.1371/journal.pone.0052416

Laura, C. (2018) *Hypoglycemia rate 'lower-than-expected' with intermittent fasting diet* Retrieved from https://diabetes.medicinematters.com/diet/lifestyle-interventions/hypoglycemia-rate-lower-than-expected-with-intermittent-fasting-/15464816

Lisa. (2018) *Glycogen depletion: Signs and symptoms.* Retrieved from https://8fit.com/fitness/glycogen-depletion-signs-symptoms-and-working-out/

Marjorie, H. (2018). *Ketosis vs. Ketoacidosis: What You Should Know.* Retrieved from https://www.healthline.com/health/ketosis-vs-ketoacidosis/

Mark, H. (2012). *Ten Reasons to Quit Your Coffee!* Retrieved from https://drhyman.com/blog/2012/06/13/ten-reasons-to-quit-your-coffee/

Mercola, J. (2011). *The exercise mistake which makes you age faster.* Retrieved from https://articles.mercola.com/sites/articles/archive/2011/06/19/innovative-revolutionary-program-to-keep-your-body-biologically-young.aspx

Mercola, J. (2013). *Should you eat before exercise?*

Retrieved from
https://fitness.mercola.com/sites/fitness/archive/2013/09/13/eating-before-exercise.aspx

Mohammad, A. *et al.* (2016) *Interferon beta overexpression attenuates adipose tissue inflammation and high fat diet-induced obesity and maintains glucose homeostasi.* Retrieved from
https://www.ncbi.nlm.nih.gov/pmc/articles/PMC5757862/

Moro, Tatiana et al. "Effects of eight weeks of time-restricted feeding (16/8) on basal metabolism, maximal strength, body composition, inflammation, and cardiovascular risk factors in resistance-trained males" *Journal of translational medicine* vol. 14,1 290. 13 Oct. 2016, doi:10.1186/s12967-016-1044-0

Nutrition Review (2013). *Medium Chain Triglycerides (MCTs).* Retrieved from
https://nutritionreview.org/2013/04/medium-chain-triglycerides-mcts/

Röjdmark, S. "Influence of Short-Term Fasting on the Pituitary-Testicular Axis in Normal Men." *Hormone Research*, U.S. National Library of Medicine, 1987, www.ncbi.nlm.nih.gov/pubmed/3106181.

Scandinavian Journal of Medicine and Science in Sports. (2018). *Effects of fasted vs fed-state exercise on performance and post-exercise metabolism: A systematic review and meta-analysis.* Retrieved from
https://www.ncbi.nlm.nih.gov/pubmed/29315892

Schwecherl, L. (2017). *21 Low-impact workouts that are more effective than you think.* Retrieved from
https://greatist.com/fitness/take-it-easy-21-unexpected-low-impact-workouts

Science Direct. (2014). *Intermittent fasting vs daily calorie restriction for type 2 diabetes prevention: A review of human findings.* Retrieved from https://www.sciencedirect.com/science/article/pii/S1931524414400200X

Sonpal, N. (2018). *How to exercise safely during intermittent fasting.* Retrieved from https://www.healthline.com/health/how-to-exercise-safely-intermittent-fasting#1

Tegan, T. (2018). *Alkaline diets: Good for your health or just another fad? Retrieved from* https://www.abc.net.au/news/health/2018-08-01/alkaline-diet-health-fact-or-fad/10055714

The British Journal of Nutrition. (2016). *Effects of aerobic exercise performed in fasted v. fed state on fat and carbohydrate metabolism in adults: A systematic review and meta-analysis.* Retrieved from https://www.ncbi.nlm.nih.gov/pubmed/27609363

Traci, M. (2018). *Why do dieters regain weight? Calorie deprivation alters body and mind, overwhelming willpower.* Retrieved from https://www.apa.org/science/about/psa/2018/05/calorie-deprivation

University of Adelaide., (2019). *Intermittent fasting could improve obese women's health.* Retrieved from https://www.sciencedaily.com/releases/2019/01/190108125526.htm

US National Library of Medicine. (2009). *Starving neurons show sex difference in autophagy.* Retrieved from https://www.ncbi.nlm.nih.gov/pmc/articles/ PMC2629091/

US National Library of Medicine. (2011). *The protein-*

retaining effects of growth hormone during fasting involve inhibition of muscle-protein breakdown. Retrieved from https://www.ncbi.nlm.nih.gov/pubmed/11147801

Walker, Cheryl, and Alicia Roberts. "Lose Fat, Preserve Muscle: Weight Training Beats Cardio for Older Adults." *Wake Forest News*, 31 Oct. 2017, news.wfu.edu/2017/10/31/lose-fat-preserve-muscle-weight-training-beats-cardio-older-adults/.

Yuri, E. (2015). *Top 12 Health Benefits of Apple Cider Vinegar You Need to Know (Backed by Science.* Retrieved from https://yurielkaim.com/health-benefits-of-apple-cider-vinegar/